2024 Edition

2 in 1 Book

PROSTATE CANCER
DIET COOKBOOK AND NUTRITION

Guide for Men Over 50

Wholesome Recipes and Expert Advice for Managing Prostate Cancer

Sawyer Jones

Copyright © Sawyer Jones, 2024.

Table of Content

Introduction

Welcome to a journey towards vibrant health and vitality! In the battle against prostate cancer, arming yourself with the right tools is paramount, and one of the most powerful weapons in your arsenal is your diet.

Picture this: You hold in your hands not just a book, but a lifeline—a comprehensive guide that marries the science of nutrition with the art of delicious cooking, specifically tailored for men over 50 navigating the complexities of prostate cancer.

But this isn't just any cookbook. This is your roadmap to reclaiming control over your health, your vitality, and your future. Gone are the days of bland, uninspiring meals that leave you feeling deprived and defeated. In their place, discover a treasure trove of flavorful, nourishing recipes designed to tantalize your taste buds while supporting your body's fight against cancer.

From hearty breakfasts that jumpstart your day to comforting dinners that warm your soul, each recipe is crafted with your well-being in mind. But this book is more than just a collection of recipes; it's your trusted companion on a holistic journey towards wellness.

So, if you're ready to harness the power of food to fuel your fight against prostate cancer, then buckle up and prepare to embark on a culinary adventure like no other. Let's dive in and discover how the right foods can not only nourish your body but also nourish your spirit as you take charge of your health and embrace life to the fullest.

Welcome to "The Prostate Cancer Diet Cookbook and Nutrition Guide for Men Over 50." Your journey starts now.

Overview of Prostate Cancer

Prostate cancer is a type of cancer that develops in the prostate gland, a small walnut-shaped gland in the male reproductive system. The prostate gland's primary function is to produce seminal fluid, which nourishes and transports sperm. Prostate cancer is one of the most common types of cancer in men, particularly in older men.

Risk Factors: Several factors can increase the risk of developing prostate cancer, including age, family history, race, and certain genetic mutations. Men over the age of 50, especially those with a family history of prostate cancer, are at higher risk.

Symptoms: In its early stages, prostate cancer may not cause any symptoms. As the cancer progresses, symptoms may include difficulty urinating, blood in the urine, erectile dysfunction, and pain in the back, hips, or pelvis.

Diagnosis: Prostate cancer is often diagnosed through a combination of physical exams, blood tests (such as the prostate-specific antigen, or PSA, test), imaging tests (such as ultrasound or MRI), and a biopsy.

Stages: Prostate cancer is staged based on the size and extent of the tumor and whether it has spread to other parts of the body. Staging helps determine the best course of treatment.

Treatment: Treatment options for prostate cancer depend on several factors, including the stage of the cancer, the patient's overall health, and personal preferences. Treatment may include active surveillance, surgery, radiation therapy, hormone therapy, chemotherapy, or a combination of these.

Prevention: While there is no guaranteed way to prevent prostate cancer, certain lifestyle changes, such as maintaining a healthy weight, eating a balanced diet, exercising regularly, and avoiding smoking, may help reduce the risk.

Importance of Diet and Nutrition in Prostate Cancer Management

Diet and nutrition play a crucial role in the management of prostate cancer. While a healthy diet cannot cure prostate cancer, it can help support overall health, strengthen the immune system, and improve quality of life during and after treatment. Here are some key ways in which diet and nutrition can impact prostate cancer:

1. Managing Treatment Side Effects: Prostate cancer treatments such as surgery, radiation therapy, and hormone therapy can cause side effects that affect appetite, digestion, and overall nutrition. A diet rich in nutrients can help manage these side effects and support the body's recovery.

2. Maintaining a Healthy Weight: Maintaining a healthy weight is important for overall health and can also improve outcomes for prostate cancer patients. Obesity has been linked to more aggressive forms of prostate cancer and poorer treatment outcomes. A balanced diet can help achieve and maintain a healthy weight.

3. Reducing Inflammation: Chronic inflammation is believed to play a role in the development and progression of prostate cancer. A diet rich in anti-inflammatory foods, such as fruits, vegetables, whole grains, and healthy fats, can help reduce inflammation in the body.

4. Supporting Immune Function: A well-balanced diet rich in vitamins, minerals, antioxidants, and other nutrients can support the immune system, helping the body fight off infections and recover from treatment more effectively.

5. Managing Hormone Levels: Some foods and dietary patterns may affect hormone levels, including testosterone, which can impact the growth and progression of prostate cancer. A diet that helps maintain healthy hormone levels may be beneficial.

6. Promoting Overall Health: A diet that is high in fruits, vegetables, whole grains, and lean proteins can help promote overall health and reduce the risk of other chronic diseases, such as heart disease and diabetes, which can impact prostate cancer outcomes.

In conclusion, while diet and nutrition cannot cure prostate cancer, they play a crucial role in supporting overall health, managing treatment side effects, and potentially improving outcomes for prostate cancer patients. A balanced diet that includes a variety of nutrient-rich foods is essential for prostate cancer management.

2. Understanding Prostate Cancer

Risk Factors for Prostate Cancer

Prostate cancer is the most common cancer in men, and several factors can increase a man's risk of developing this disease. While some risk factors, such as age and family history, cannot be changed, understanding these risk factors can help men make informed decisions about their health and screening options. Here are some key risk factors for prostate cancer:

1. Age: The risk of developing prostate cancer increases with age. Prostate cancer is rare in men under 40 but becomes more common as men get older. The majority of prostate cancers are diagnosed in men over the age of 65.

2. Family History: Men with a family history of prostate cancer are at higher risk. Having a father, brother, or son with prostate cancer doubles a man's risk of developing the disease. The risk is even higher if multiple family members are affected or if the cancer was diagnosed at a young age.

3. Race: Prostate cancer occurs more frequently in African American men than in men of other races. African American men are also more likely to be diagnosed at an advanced stage and have a higher risk of dying from prostate cancer.

4. Genetic Factors: Certain inherited genetic mutations, such as mutations in the BRCA1 or BRCA2 genes, may increase the risk of developing prostate cancer. These mutations are also associated with an increased risk of other cancers, such as breast and ovarian cancer.

5. Dietary Factors: Some studies suggest that a diet high in red meat or high-fat dairy products and low in fruits and vegetables may increase the risk of prostate cancer. However, more research is needed to fully understand the relationship between diet and prostate cancer risk.

6. Obesity: Obesity has been linked to an increased risk of developing more aggressive forms of prostate cancer and a higher risk of cancer recurrence after treatment.

7. Smoking: Some studies suggest that smoking may increase the risk of developing aggressive prostate cancer. Smoking is also a risk factor for many other cancers and other serious health conditions.

8. Exposure to Certain Chemicals: Some studies suggest that exposure to certain chemicals, such as Agent Orange, may increase the risk of developing prostate cancer. However, more research is needed in this area.

It's important to note that having one or more risk factors does not mean that a man will definitely develop prostate cancer. Many men with one or more risk factors never develop the disease, while some men with no known risk factors do. Regular screening and early detection are key to managing prostate cancer risk.

Stages and Types of Prostate Cancer

Prostate cancer is typically staged based on the extent of the disease, including the size of the tumor and whether it has spread to other parts of the body. Staging helps doctors determine the best treatment approach and predict the likely outcome of the disease. Prostate cancer can also be classified into different types based on how the cancer cells look under a microscope. Here are the stages and types of prostate cancer:

Stages of Prostate Cancer:

1. Stage I: The cancer is small and confined to the prostate gland. It is usually slow-growing and may not cause symptoms.

2. Stage II: The cancer is still confined to the prostate gland but may be larger than in Stage I. It may be detected during a biopsy or imaging tests.

3. Stage III: The cancer has spread beyond the prostate gland to nearby tissues, such as the seminal vesicles. It may also be detected in lymph nodes near the prostate.

4. Stage IV: The cancer has spread to distant parts of the body, such as the bones, liver, or lungs. This is known as metastatic prostate cancer and is more difficult to treat.

Types of Prostate Cancer:

1. Adenocarcinoma: This is the most common type of prostate cancer, accounting for about 99% of cases. It starts in the gland cells of the prostate and usually grows slowly.

2. Small Cell Carcinoma: This is a rare and aggressive type of prostate cancer that tends to grow and spread quickly. It is less common than adenocarcinoma.

3. Transitional Cell (or Urothelial) Carcinoma: This type of prostate cancer begins in the cells that line the bladder and can spread to the prostate. It is also rare.

4. Sarcomas, Carcinoid Tumors, and Other Rare Types: These are rare types of prostate cancer that develop in the connective tissues or neuroendocrine cells of the prostate.

Understanding the stage and type of prostate cancer is essential for determining the most appropriate treatment plan. Treatment options may include surgery, radiation therapy, hormone therapy, chemotherapy, or a combination of these. Early detection through regular screening is crucial for improving the chances of successful treatment and survival.

Common Treatments and Side Effects of Prostate Cancer

Prostate cancer treatment is highly individualized and depends on several factors, including the stage and aggressiveness of the cancer, as well as the patient's overall health and preferences. Here are some common treatments and their associated side effects:

1. Active Surveillance: For some men with low-risk prostate cancer, active surveillance may be recommended. This involves closely monitoring the cancer with regular PSA tests, digital rectal exams, and possibly imaging tests. Treatment is only started if the cancer shows signs of progressing.

2. Surgery (Prostatectomy): Surgery to remove the prostate gland (prostatectomy) is a common treatment for prostate cancer. Side effects can include urinary incontinence, erectile dysfunction, and infertility.

3. Radiation Therapy: Radiation therapy uses high-energy rays to kill cancer cells. Side effects can include fatigue, urinary problems, bowel problems, and erectile dysfunction.

4. Hormone Therapy: Hormone therapy, also known as androgen deprivation therapy (ADT), works by reducing the levels of male hormones (androgens) in the body, which can help slow the growth of prostate cancer. Side effects can include hot flashes, fatigue, loss of muscle mass, and erectile dysfunction.

5. Chemotherapy: Chemotherapy uses drugs to kill cancer cells. It is typically used in advanced prostate cancer that has spread to other parts of the body. Side effects can include nausea, hair loss, fatigue, and increased risk of infections.

6. Immunotherapy: Immunotherapy uses drugs to stimulate the immune system to recognize and attack cancer cells. Side effects can include fatigue, flu-like symptoms, and skin reactions.

7. Targeted Therapy: Targeted therapy uses drugs that target specific molecules involved in cancer growth. Side effects can vary depending on the drug used.

8. Bone-Directed Therapy: Prostate cancer that has spread to the bones may be treated with bone-directed therapy to help reduce pain and the risk of fractures. Side effects can include nausea, diarrhea, and fatigue.

It's important for patients to discuss potential side effects with their healthcare team and to report any side effects they experience during treatment. Many side effects can be managed with medications, lifestyle changes, or other treatments. Maintaining open communication with healthcare providers can help ensure that patients receive the best possible care and support throughout their treatment journey.

3. The Role of Diet in Prostate Cancer Prevention

- Key Nutrients for Prostate Health

Diet plays a significant role in prostate cancer prevention. While no single food or nutrient can prevent prostate cancer, a healthy diet that includes a variety of nutrient-rich foods may help reduce the risk. Here are some key nutrients for prostate health that can be included in a balanced diet:

1. Selenium: Selenium is a mineral with antioxidant properties that may help protect prostate cells from damage. Good food sources of selenium include Brazil nuts, seafood (such as tuna and shrimp), whole grains, and sunflower seeds.

2. Vitamin E: Vitamin E is another antioxidant that may help protect prostate cells. Foods rich in vitamin E include nuts (such as almonds and hazelnuts), seeds (such as sunflower seeds), spinach, and broccoli.

3. Lycopene: Lycopene is a powerful antioxidant that gives fruits and vegetables their red color. Some studies suggest that lycopene may help reduce the risk of prostate cancer. Good sources of lycopene include tomatoes, watermelon, and pink grapefruit.

4. Zinc: Zinc is a mineral that is important for prostate health. It is involved in the production of prostate fluid and may help reduce the risk of developing prostate cancer. Good sources of zinc include oysters, red meat, poultry, beans, and nuts.

5. Omega-3 Fatty Acids: Omega-3 fatty acids are healthy fats that may help reduce inflammation in the body. Some studies suggest that omega-3 fatty acids may help reduce the risk of developing prostate cancer. Good sources of omega-3 fatty acids include fatty fish (such as salmon, mackerel, and sardines), flaxseeds, and walnuts.

6. Vitamin D: Vitamin D is important for overall health and may also play a role in prostate health. Some studies suggest that vitamin D deficiency may be linked to an increased risk of developing prostate cancer. Good sources of vitamin D include fatty fish, egg yolks, and fortified foods (such as milk and cereal).

Including these key nutrients in your diet, along with a variety of fruits, vegetables, whole grains, and healthy fats, can help support prostate health and reduce the risk of developing prostate cancer. It's also important to maintain a healthy weight, exercise regularly, and avoid smoking for overall prostate health.

- Foods to Include and Avoid

Foods to Include:

1. Fruits: Berries, apples, oranges, and grapes.
2. Vegetables: Spinach, kale, broccoli, and Brussels sprouts.
3. Whole Grains: Oats, brown rice, quinoa, and whole wheat bread.
4. Healthy Fats: Avocado, olive oil, nuts (like almonds, walnuts), and seeds (such as flaxseeds, chia seeds).
5. Fish: Salmon, sardines, trout, and mackerel.
6. Soy Products: Tofu, tempeh, edamame, and soy milk.
7. Legumes: Lentils, chickpeas, black beans, and kidney beans.
8. Herbs and Spices: Turmeric, ginger, garlic, and cinnamon.

Foods to Avoid:

1. Red and Processed Meats: Beef, lamb, pork, and processed meats like bacon, sausage, and deli meats.
2. High-Fat Dairy: Full-fat milk, cheese, and cream.
3. Saturated and Trans Fats: Fried foods, fast food, and commercially baked goods.
4. Excessive Calcium: Avoid calcium supplements and limit intake of high-calcium foods like dairy.

5. Excessive Alcohol: Limit alcohol consumption, especially beer and spirits.

General Tips:

- Choose lean protein sources like chicken, turkey, and fish over red meat.
- Opt for whole grains over refined grains.
- Use healthy fats like olive oil and avocado instead of butter or margarine.
- Include a variety of fruits and vegetables in your diet for maximum nutrition.
- Drink plenty of water and limit sugary drinks and sodas.

These dietary recommendations, along with a healthy lifestyle that includes regular exercise and maintaining a healthy weight, can help support prostate health and reduce the risk of developing prostate cancer.

4. Nutrition Strategies During Prostate Cancer Treatment

- Managing Side Effects of Treatment Through Diet

Prostate cancer treatment can often cause side effects that affect a man's appetite, digestion, and overall nutrition. Managing these side effects through diet can help improve quality of life and support the body's recovery. Here are some nutrition strategies to consider during prostate cancer treatment:

1. Managing Digestive Issues:
   - Eat Small, Frequent Meals: Eating smaller meals throughout the day can be easier on the digestive system.
   - Avoid Gas-Producing Foods: Limiting foods that can cause gas, such as beans, broccoli, and cabbage, may help reduce bloating and discomfort.
   - Stay Hydrated: Drink plenty of fluids, but avoid carbonated drinks, which can cause gas.

2. Dealing with Changes in Taste and Smell:
   - Experiment with Flavors: Try using herbs, spices, and marinades to enhance the flavor of foods.
   - Cold Foods: Cold foods may have less aroma and may be more tolerable if taste and smell changes are an issue.

3. Managing Nausea:
   - Eat Plain Foods: Bland, easy-to-digest foods like crackers, rice, and bananas may help settle the stomach.
   - Avoid Strong Smells: Strong odors can trigger nausea, so try to avoid cooking or being around foods with strong smells.

4. Maintaining Weight:
   - Focus on Nutrient-Dense Foods: Choose foods that are high in nutrients and calories to help maintain weight.

- Include Protein: Protein-rich foods like lean meats, fish, eggs, and legumes can help preserve muscle mass.

5. Coping with Fatigue:
  - Eat Light Meals: Eating smaller, more frequent meals may be easier when energy levels are low.
  - Stay Hydrated: Dehydration can worsen fatigue, so be sure to drink plenty of fluids.

6. Managing Diarrhea:
  - Avoid High-Fiber Foods: Foods high in fiber, such as raw vegetables, whole grains, and beans, may worsen diarrhea.
  - Stay Hydrated: Diarrhea can lead to dehydration, so it's important to drink plenty of fluids.

7. Addressing Constipation:
  - Increase Fiber Intake: Foods high in fiber, such as fruits, vegetables, and whole grains, can help relieve constipation.
  - Stay Hydrated: Drinking plenty of fluids can also help prevent constipation.

8. Hydration:
  - Drink Plenty of Fluids: Staying hydrated is important for overall health and can help manage many side effects of treatment.

9. Individualized Approach:
  - Consult with a Dietitian: A registered dietitian can help create a personalized nutrition plan based on individual needs and treatment side effects.

Managing side effects through diet during prostate cancer treatment is an important aspect of overall care. By making thoughtful food choices and adopting strategies to address specific side effects, men undergoing treatment can support their body's healing process and improve their quality of life.

- Maintaining a Healthy Weight

Maintaining a healthy weight is important for overall health and can also impact the risk of developing prostate cancer and the outcomes of treatment. Here are some tips for maintaining a healthy weight:

1. Balanced Diet: Focus on eating a balanced diet that includes a variety of fruits, vegetables, whole grains, and lean proteins. Limit the intake of processed foods, sugary drinks, and high-fat foods.

2. Portion Control: Pay attention to portion sizes and avoid eating larger portions than you need. Use smaller plates and bowls to help control portion sizes.

3. Regular Exercise: Engage in regular physical activity to help maintain a healthy weight. Aim for at least 150 minutes of moderate-intensity exercise per week, such as brisk walking, cycling, or swimming.

4. Strength Training: Incorporate strength training exercises into your routine to help build muscle mass, which can increase metabolism and support weight management.

5. Stay Hydrated: Drink plenty of water throughout the day to stay hydrated and avoid confusing thirst with hunger.

6. Monitor Your Weight: Regularly weigh yourself and keep track of your weight to monitor changes over time. This can help you make adjustments to your diet and exercise routine as needed.

7. Seek Support: If you're struggling to maintain a healthy weight, consider seeking support from a healthcare provider, dietitian, or support group. They can provide guidance and encouragement to help you reach your goals.

Maintaining a healthy weight is just one aspect of overall health, but it can have a significant impact on your well-being and reduce the risk of developing prostate cancer. By following these tips and making healthy lifestyle choices, you can support your weight management goals and improve your overall health.

5. Breakfast Recipes

1. Avocado Toast with Eggs

Ingredients:
- 2 slices whole grain bread
- 1 ripe avocado
- 2 eggs
- Salt and pepper to taste

Prep Time: 5 minutes
Cooking Time: 10 minutes

Instructions:
1. Toast the bread until golden brown.
2. Mash the avocado and spread it evenly on the toast.
3. Cook the eggs to your liking (e.g., scrambled, fried, or poached) and place them on top of the avocado.
4. Season with salt and pepper.

Nutritional Information:
- Calories: 350
- Protein: 15g
- Carbohydrates: 28g
- Fat: 20g

---

2. Greek Yogurt Parfait

Ingredients:
- 1 cup Greek yogurt
- 1/2 cup granola
- 1/2 cup mixed berries (e.g., strawberries, blueberries, raspberries)

Prep Time: 5 minutes
Cooking Time: 0 minutes

Instructions:
1. In a bowl or glass, layer Greek yogurt, granola, and mixed berries.
2. Repeat the layers until all ingredients are used up.

Nutritional Information:
- Calories: 300
- Protein: 20g
- Carbohydrates: 40g
- Fat: 8g

---

3. Veggie Omelette

Ingredients:
- 2 eggs
- 1/4 cup chopped bell peppers
- 1/4 cup chopped onions
- 1/4 cup chopped spinach
- Salt and pepper to taste
- 1 tsp olive oil

Prep Time: 5 minutes
Cooking Time: 10 minutes

Instructions:
1. In a bowl, whisk the eggs with salt and pepper.
2. Heat olive oil in a pan over medium heat.
3. Add the bell peppers, onions, and spinach to the pan and sauté until softened.
4. Pour the eggs over the vegetables and cook until the eggs are set.
5. Fold the omelette in half and serve.

Nutritional Information:
- Calories: 250
- Protein: 16g
- Carbohydrates: 10g
- Fat: 15g

---

4. Overnight Oats

Ingredients:
- 1/2 cup rolled oats
- 1/2 cup almond milk
- 1 tbsp chia seeds
- 1/2 tsp vanilla extract
- 1/2 banana, sliced
- 1 tbsp honey

Prep Time: 5 minutes
Cooking Time: 0 minutes

Instructions:
1. In a jar or container, combine oats, almond milk, chia seeds, and vanilla extract.
2. Stir well, cover, and refrigerate overnight.
3. In the morning, top with sliced banana and drizzle with honey.

Nutritional Information:
- Calories: 350
- Protein: 10g
- Carbohydrates: 60g
- Fat: 8g

---

5. Whole Grain Pancakes

Ingredients:
- 1/2 cup whole wheat flour
- 1/2 cup oat flour
- 1 tsp baking powder
- 1/2 tsp cinnamon
- 1/2 cup almond milk
- 1 egg
- 1 tbsp honey
- 1/2 tsp vanilla extract

Prep Time: 10 minutes
Cooking Time: 15 minutes

Instructions:
1. In a bowl, whisk together the flours, baking powder, and cinnamon.
2. In another bowl, whisk together the almond milk, egg, honey, and vanilla extract.
3. Pour the wet ingredients into the dry ingredients and mix until well combined.
4. Heat a non-stick pan over medium heat and lightly grease with cooking spray.
5. Pour 1/4 cup of batter onto the pan for each pancake and cook until bubbles form on the surface.
6. Flip the pancakes and cook for another minute or until golden brown.

Nutritional Information:
- Calories: 300
- Protein: 10g
- Carbohydrates: 50g
- Fat: 7g

---

6. Breakfast Burrito

Ingredients:
- 2 eggs
- 2 whole grain tortillas
- 1/4 cup black beans, drained and rinsed
- 1/4 cup diced tomatoes
- 1/4 cup diced bell peppers
- 1/4 cup shredded cheddar cheese
- Salt and pepper to taste
- 1 tsp olive oil

Prep Time: 5 minutes
Cooking Time: 10 minutes

Instructions:
1. In a bowl, whisk the eggs with salt and pepper.
2. Heat olive oil in a pan over medium heat.
3. Add the eggs to the pan and scramble until cooked through.
4. Place the tortillas on a plate and top each with half of the scrambled eggs, black beans, tomatoes, bell peppers, and cheese.
5. Roll up the tortillas to form burritos.

Nutritional Information:
- Calories: 400
- Protein: 20g
- Carbohydrates: 30g
- Fat: 20g

---

7. Peanut Butter Banana Smoothie

Ingredients:
- 1 banana

- 1 tbsp peanut butter
- 1/2 cup Greek yogurt
- 1/2 cup almond milk
- 1 tbsp honey
- Ice cubes (optional)

Prep Time: 5 minutes
Cooking Time: 0 minutes

Instructions:
1. In a blender, combine the banana, peanut butter, Greek yogurt, almond milk, honey, and ice cubes.
2. Blend until smooth and creamy.

Nutritional Information:
- Calories: 350
- Protein: 15g
- Carbohydrates: 40g
- Fat: 15g

---

8. Chia Seed Breakfast Bowl

Ingredients:
- 1/4 cup chia seeds
- 1 cup almond milk
- 1/2 tsp vanilla extract
- 1 tbsp honey
- 1/4 cup mixed berries
- 1 tbsp sliced almonds

Prep Time: 5 minutes
Cooking Time: 0 minutes

Instructions:
1. In a bowl, combine chia seeds, almond milk, vanilla extract, and honey. Stir well.
2. Cover and refrigerate overnight, or for at least 2 hours, until the mixture thickens.
3. In the morning, top with mixed berries and sliced almonds.

Nutritional Information:
- Calories: 300
- Protein: 10g
- Carbohydrates: 30g
- Fat: 15g

---

9. Spinach and Feta Breakfast Wrap

Ingredients:
- 1 whole grain tortilla
- 2 eggs, scrambled
- 1/4 cup cooked spinach
- 2 tbsp crumbled feta cheese
- Salt and pepper to taste

Prep Time: 5 minutes
Cooking Time: 5 minutes

Instructions:
1. Place the tortilla on a plate and top with scrambled eggs, cooked spinach, and feta cheese.
2. Season with salt and pepper.
3. Roll up the tortilla to form a wrap.

Nutritional Information:
- Calories: 350

- Protein: 20g
- Carbohydrates: 25g
- Fat: 18g

---

10. Banana Oat Pancakes

Ingredients:
- 1/2 cup rolled oats
- 1 ripe banana
- 1/2 cup almond milk
- 1 egg
- 1/2 tsp cinnamon
- 1/2 tsp vanilla extract
- Cooking spray

Prep Time: 5 minutes
Cooking Time: 10 minutes

Instructions:
1. In a blender, combine oats, banana, almond milk, egg, cinnamon, and vanilla extract. Blend until smooth.
2. Heat a non-stick pan over medium heat and lightly grease with cooking spray.
3. Pour 1/4 cup of batter onto the pan for each pancake.
4. Cook for 2-3 minutes per side, or until golden brown.

Nutritional Information:
- Calories: 300
- Protein: 10g
- Carbohydrates: 45g
- Fat: 8g

---

11. Apple Cinnamon Baked Oatmeal

Ingredients:
- 1 cup rolled oats
- 1 apple, diced
- 1/2 tsp cinnamon
- 1/2 tsp baking powder
- 1/4 cup almond milk
- 1 egg
- 1 tbsp maple syrup
- 1 tbsp chopped walnuts (optional)

Prep Time: 10 minutes
Cooking Time: 25 minutes

Instructions:
1. Preheat the oven to 350°F (175°C) and grease a baking dish.
2. In a bowl, combine oats, apple, cinnamon, and baking powder.
3. In another bowl, whisk together almond milk, egg, and maple syrup.
4. Pour the wet ingredients into the dry ingredients and mix until well combined.
5. Pour the mixture into the baking dish and sprinkle with chopped walnuts.
6. Bake for 25 minutes, or until set and golden brown.

Nutritional Information:
- Calories: 300
- Protein: 10g
- Carbohydrates: 45g
- Fat: 8g

---

12. Smoked Salmon and Cream Cheese Bagel

Ingredients:
- 1 whole grain bagel, sliced and toasted
- 2 tbsp cream cheese
- 2 oz smoked salmon
- 1/4 cup sliced cucumber
- 1 tbsp chopped chives

Prep Time: 5 minutes
Cooking Time: 0 minutes

Instructions:
1. Spread cream cheese on each half of the bagel.
2. Top with smoked salmon, cucumber slices, and chopped chives.
3. Serve open-faced.

Nutritional Information:
- Calories: 350
- Protein: 20g
- Carbohydrates: 40g
- Fat: 12g

---

13. Blueberry Almond Butter Smoothie

Ingredients:
- 1/2 cup blueberries
- 1 banana
- 2 tbsp almond butter
- 1/2 cup Greek yogurt
- 1/2 cup almond milk
- Ice cubes (optional)

Prep Time: 5 minutes
Cooking Time: 0 minutes

Instructions:
1. In a blender, combine blueberries, banana, almond butter, Greek yogurt, almond milk, and ice cubes.
2. Blend until smooth and creamy.

Nutritional Information:
- Calories: 350
- Protein: 15g
- Carbohydrates: 40g
- Fat: 15g

---

14. Breakfast Quinoa Bowl

Ingredients:
- 1/2 cup cooked quinoa
- 1/2 cup almond milk
- 1/2 tsp cinnamon
- 1/2 banana, sliced
- 1 tbsp chopped nuts (e.g., almonds, walnuts)
- 1 tbsp honey

Prep Time: 5 minutes
Cooking Time: 10 minutes

Instructions:
1. In a saucepan, combine quinoa, almond milk, and cinnamon. Cook over medium heat until heated through.
2. Transfer the quinoa to a bowl and top with banana slices, chopped nuts, and honey.

Nutritional Information:
- Calories: 300
- Protein: 10g
- Carbohydrates: 45g
- Fat: 8g

---

15. Breakfast Tacos

Ingredients:
- 2 corn tortillas
- 2 eggs, scrambled
- 1/4 cup black beans, drained and rinsed
- 1/4 cup diced tomatoes
- 1/4 cup diced avocado
- 1 tbsp chopped cilantro
- Salt and pepper to taste

Prep Time: 5 minutes
Cooking Time: 10 minutes

Instructions:
1. Heat the tortillas in a dry skillet over medium heat until warm.
2. Fill each tortilla with scrambled eggs, black beans, tomatoes, avocado, and cilantro.
3. Season with salt and pepper.

Nutritional Information:
- Calories: 350
- Protein: 20g
- Carbohydrates: 30g
- Fat: 18g

---

6. Lunch Recipes

1. Grilled Salmon Salad

Ingredients:
- 4 oz grilled salmon
- 2 cups mixed greens
- 1/2 cucumber, sliced
- 1/4 cup cherry tomatoes, halved
- 1/4 cup red onion, thinly sliced
- 1/4 avocado, sliced
- 1 tbsp olive oil
- 1 tbsp lemon juice
- Salt and pepper to taste

Instructions:
1. In a large bowl, combine mixed greens, cucumber, cherry tomatoes, and red onion.
2. Top with grilled salmon and avocado slices.
3. Drizzle with olive oil and lemon juice. Season with salt and pepper.

Nutritional Information:
- Calories: 400
- Protein: 30g
- Carbohydrates: 15g
- Fat: 25g

---

2. Quinoa and Black Bean Bowl

Ingredients:
- 1/2 cup cooked quinoa
- 1/2 cup black beans, drained and rinsed
- 1/4 cup corn kernels

- 1/4 cup diced bell peppers
- 1/4 cup diced tomatoes
- 1/4 avocado, sliced
- 1 tbsp chopped cilantro
- 1 tbsp lime juice
- Salt and pepper to taste

Instructions:
1. In a bowl, combine cooked quinoa, black beans, corn, bell peppers, and tomatoes.
2. Top with avocado slices and chopped cilantro.
3. Drizzle with lime juice. Season with salt and pepper.

Nutritional Information:
- Calories: 350
- Protein: 15g
- Carbohydrates: 50g
- Fat: 10g

---

3. Turkey and Hummus Wrap

Ingredients:
- 1 whole grain wrap
- 3 oz sliced turkey breast
- 2 tbsp hummus
- 1/4 cup shredded carrots
- 1/4 cup baby spinach leaves
- 1/4 cup cucumber, thinly sliced

Instructions:
1. Spread hummus evenly over the wrap.
2. Layer turkey breast, shredded carrots, spinach leaves, and cucumber slices.

3. Roll up the wrap and slice in half.

Nutritional Information:
- Calories: 350
- Protein: 25g
- Carbohydrates: 35g
- Fat: 12g

---

4. Lentil and Vegetable Soup

Ingredients:
- 1/2 cup dried lentils
- 2 cups vegetable broth
- 1/2 cup diced carrots
- 1/2 cup diced celery
- 1/2 cup diced onion
- 1 garlic clove, minced
- 1/2 tsp cumin
- Salt and pepper to taste

Instructions:
1. In a pot, combine lentils, vegetable broth, carrots, celery, onion, garlic, and cumin.
2. Bring to a boil, then reduce heat and simmer for 20-25 minutes, or until lentils are tender.
3. Season with salt and pepper.

Nutritional Information:
- Calories: 300
- Protein: 18g
- Carbohydrates: 50g
- Fat: 2g

---

5. Chickpea Salad Sandwich

Ingredients:
- 1/2 cup canned chickpeas, drained and rinsed
- 1 tbsp Greek yogurt
- 1 tsp Dijon mustard
- 1/4 cup diced red bell pepper
- 1/4 cup diced cucumber
- 1 tbsp chopped parsley
- Salt and pepper to taste
- 2 slices whole grain bread

Instructions:
1. In a bowl, mash the chickpeas with a fork.
2. Stir in Greek yogurt, Dijon mustard, red bell pepper, cucumber, parsley, salt, and pepper.
3. Spread the mixture onto one slice of bread and top with the other slice.

Nutritional Information:
- Calories: 350
- Protein: 15g
- Carbohydrates: 60g
- Fat: 5g

---

6. Roasted Vegetable Quinoa Salad

Ingredients:
- 1/2 cup cooked quinoa
- 1/2 cup roasted vegetables (e.g., bell peppers, zucchini, eggplant)
- 2 tbsp crumbled feta cheese
- 1 tbsp chopped walnuts

- 1 tbsp balsamic vinegar
- 1 tsp olive oil
- Salt and pepper to taste

Instructions:
1. In a bowl, combine cooked quinoa, roasted vegetables, feta cheese, and walnuts.
2. Drizzle with balsamic vinegar and olive oil. Season with salt and pepper.

Nutritional Information:
- Calories: 350
- Protein: 12g
- Carbohydrates: 40g
- Fat: 15g

---

7. Tuna Salad Stuffed Avocado

Ingredients:
- 1 can tuna, drained
- 1/4 cup Greek yogurt
- 1/4 cup diced celery
- 1/4 cup diced red onion
- 1 tbsp lemon juice
- 2 avocados, halved and pitted
- Salt and pepper to taste

Instructions:
1. In a bowl, combine tuna, Greek yogurt, celery, red onion, lemon juice, salt, and pepper.
2. Spoon the tuna salad into the avocado halves.

Nutritional Information:
- Calories: 350

- Protein: 25g
- Carbohydrates: 15g
- Fat: 20g

---

8. Chicken and Vegetable Stir-Fry

Ingredients:
- 4 oz chicken breast, sliced
- 1 cup mixed vegetables (e.g., bell peppers, broccoli, carrots)
- 1/4 cup sliced mushrooms
- 2 tbsp soy sauce
- 1 tbsp hoisin sauce
- 1 tsp sesame oil
- 1/2 tsp minced garlic
- Cooked brown rice

Instructions:
1. In a pan, heat sesame oil over medium heat.
2. Add chicken and cook until browned.
3. Add vegetables, mushrooms, soy sauce, hoisin sauce, and garlic. Cook until vegetables are tender.
4. Serve over cooked brown rice.

Nutritional Information:
- Calories: 400
- Protein: 30g
- Carbohydrates: 40g
- Fat: 15g

---

9. Turkey and Cranberry Wrap

Ingredients:
- 1 whole grain wrap
- 3 oz sliced turkey breast
- 2 tbsp cranberry sauce
- 1/4 cup baby spinach leaves
- 1/4 cup shredded carrots

Instructions:
1. Spread cranberry sauce evenly over the wrap.
2. Layer turkey breast, baby spinach leaves, and shredded carrots.
3. Roll up the wrap and slice in half.

Nutritional Information:
- Calories: 350
- Protein: 25g
- Carbohydrates: 35g
- Fat: 12g

---

10. Lentil and Spinach Soup

Ingredients:
- 1/2 cup dried lentils
- 2 cups vegetable broth
- 1/2 cup diced carrots
- 1/2 cup diced celery
- 1/2 cup diced onion
- 1 garlic clove, minced
- 1/2 tsp cumin
- 1/2 cup chopped spinach
- Salt and pepper to taste

Instructions:
1. In a pot, combine lentils, vegetable broth, carrots, celery, onion, garlic, and cumin.
2. Bring to a boil, then reduce heat and simmer for 20-25 minutes, or until lentils are tender.
3. Stir in chopped spinach and cook for an additional 5 minutes.
4. Season with salt and pepper.

Nutritional Information:
- Calories: 300
- Protein: 18g
- Carbohydrates: 50g
- Fat: 2g

---

11. Egg Salad Sandwich

Ingredients:
- 2 hard-boiled eggs, chopped
- 2 tbsp Greek yogurt
- 1 tsp Dijon mustard
- 1/4 cup diced celery
- 1/4 cup diced red onion
- Salt and pepper to taste
- 2 slices whole grain bread

Instructions:
1. In a bowl, combine chopped hard-boiled eggs, Greek yogurt, Dijon mustard, celery, red onion, salt, and pepper.
2. Spread the mixture onto one slice of bread and top with the other slice.

Nutritional Information:
- Calories: 350
- Protein: 20g

- Carbohydrates: 35g
- Fat: 15g

---

12. Vegetable and Bean Chili

Ingredients:
- 1 can black beans, drained and rinsed
- 1 can kidney beans, drained and rinsed
- 1 can diced tomatoes
- 1 cup vegetable broth
- 1/2 cup diced onion
- 1/2 cup diced bell peppers
- 1/2 cup corn kernels
- 1/2 tsp chili powder
- 1/2 tsp cumin
- Salt and pepper to taste

Instructions:
1. In a pot, combine black beans, kidney beans, diced tomatoes, vegetable broth, onion, bell peppers, corn, chili powder, cumin, salt, and pepper.
2. Bring to a boil, then reduce heat and simmer for 20-25 minutes.
3. Serve hot.

Nutritional Information:
- Calories: 350
- Protein: 20g
- Carbohydrates: 60g
- Fat: 2g

---

13. Sweet Potato and Black Bean Tacos

Ingredients:
- 2 small sweet potatoes, peeled and diced
- 1 can (15 oz) black beans, drained and rinsed
- 1 tsp chili powder
- 1/2 tsp cumin
- 1/2 tsp garlic powder
- Salt and pepper to taste
- 8 small corn tortillas
- Optional toppings: avocado slices, salsa, cilantro, lime wedges

Instructions:
1. Preheat the oven to 400°F (200°C).
2. Place the diced sweet potatoes on a baking sheet and drizzle with olive oil. Sprinkle with chili powder, cumin, garlic powder, salt, and pepper. Toss to coat.
3. Roast the sweet potatoes in the oven for 20-25 minutes, or until tender and slightly caramelized.
4. In a small saucepan, heat the black beans over medium heat. Season with salt and pepper.
5. Heat the corn tortillas in a dry skillet over medium heat until warmed.
6. To assemble the tacos, place a spoonful of black beans on each tortilla, followed by the roasted sweet potatoes. Top with avocado slices, salsa, cilantro, and a squeeze of lime juice.

Nutritional Information:
- Calories: 350
- Protein: 10g
- Carbohydrates: 60g
- Fat: 5g

—

14. Chicken and Vegetable Stir-Fry

Ingredients:
- 1 tbsp olive oil
- 1 lb chicken breast, thinly sliced
- 2 cups mixed vegetables (e.g., bell peppers, broccoli, snap peas, carrots)
- 2 cloves garlic, minced
- 2 tbsp soy sauce
- 1 tbsp hoisin sauce
- 1 tsp sesame oil
- Cooked brown rice, for serving

Instructions:
1. Heat the olive oil in a large skillet or wok over medium-high heat.
2. Add the sliced chicken breast and cook until browned and cooked through.
3. Add the mixed vegetables and garlic to the skillet. Cook, stirring frequently, until the vegetables are tender-crisp.
4. In a small bowl, whisk together the soy sauce, hoisin sauce, and sesame oil. Pour the sauce over the chicken and vegetables in the skillet. Stir to coat.
5. Serve the chicken and vegetable stir-fry over cooked brown rice.

Nutritional Information:
- Calories: 400
- Protein: 35g
- Carbohydrates: 40g
- Fat: 10g

---

15. Lentil and Spinach Soup

Ingredients:
- 1 tbsp olive oil

- 1 onion, chopped
- 2 carrots, diced
- 2 celery stalks, diced
- 2 cloves garlic, minced
- 1 tsp cumin
- 1/2 tsp smoked paprika
- 1 cup dried green lentils, rinsed and drained
- 6 cups vegetable broth
- 4 cups fresh spinach
- Salt and pepper to taste
- Lemon wedges, for serving

Instructions:
1. Heat the olive oil in a large pot over medium heat. Add the onion, carrots, and celery. Cook, stirring occasionally, until the vegetables are softened.
2. Add the garlic, cumin, and smoked paprika to the pot. Cook, stirring constantly, for 1 minute.
3. Add the lentils and vegetable broth to the pot. Bring to a boil, then reduce heat and simmer for 20-25 minutes, or until the lentils are tender.
4. Stir in the fresh spinach and cook until wilted. Season with salt and pepper.
5. Serve the lentil and spinach soup with lemon wedges for squeezing.

Nutritional Information:
- Calories: 350
- Protein: 20g
- Carbohydrates: 55g
- Fat: 5g

---

7. Dinner Recipes

1. Grilled Chicken Breast with Quinoa Salad

Ingredients:
- 4 boneless, skinless chicken breasts
- 1 tbsp olive oil
- 1 tsp garlic powder
- 1 tsp smoked paprika
- Salt and pepper to taste
- 1 cup cooked quinoa
- 1/2 cup cherry tomatoes, halved
- 1/2 cup cucumber, diced
- 1/4 cup red onion, thinly sliced
- 2 tbsp chopped fresh parsley
- 2 tbsp lemon juice
- 1 tbsp olive oil

Instructions:
1. Preheat grill to medium-high heat.
2. Rub chicken breasts with olive oil and season with garlic powder, smoked paprika, salt, and pepper.
3. Grill chicken breasts for 6-7 minutes per side, or until cooked through.
4. In a large bowl, combine cooked quinoa, cherry tomatoes, cucumber, red onion, parsley, lemon juice, and olive oil. Season with salt and pepper.
5. Serve grilled chicken breasts with quinoa salad on the side.

Nutritional Information:
- Calories: 400
- Protein: 40g
- Carbohydrates: 30g
- Fat: 15g

---

2. Baked Salmon with Roasted Vegetables

Ingredients:
- 4 salmon fillets
- 1 tbsp olive oil
- 1 tsp garlic powder
- 1 tsp dried thyme
- Salt and pepper to taste
- 2 cups mixed vegetables (e.g., bell peppers, zucchini, cherry tomatoes)
- 1 tbsp balsamic vinegar
- 1 tsp honey
- 1/2 tsp Dijon mustard

Instructions:
1. Preheat oven to 400°F (200°C).
2. Place salmon fillets on a baking sheet lined with parchment paper. Drizzle with olive oil and sprinkle with garlic powder, dried thyme, salt, and pepper.
3. In a bowl, toss mixed vegetables with balsamic vinegar, honey, Dijon mustard, salt, and pepper. Spread vegetables on a separate baking sheet lined with parchment paper.
4. Bake salmon and vegetables in the preheated oven for 15-20 minutes, or until salmon is cooked through and vegetables are tender.
5. Serve baked salmon with roasted vegetables.

Nutritional Information:
- Calories: 350
- Protein: 30g
- Carbohydrates: 15g
- Fat: 20g

—

3. Turkey and Vegetable Stir-Fry

Ingredients:
- 1 tbsp olive oil
- 1 lb ground turkey
- 2 cups mixed vegetables (e.g., bell peppers, broccoli, snap peas, carrots)
- 2 cloves garlic, minced
- 2 tbsp soy sauce
- 1 tbsp hoisin sauce
- 1 tsp sesame oil
- Cooked brown rice, for serving

Instructions:
1. Heat olive oil in a large skillet or wok over medium-high heat.
2. Add ground turkey and cook until browned and cooked through.
3. Add mixed vegetables and garlic to the skillet. Cook, stirring frequently, until vegetables are tender-crisp.
4. In a small bowl, whisk together soy sauce, hoisin sauce, and sesame oil. Pour sauce over turkey and vegetables. Stir to combine.
5. Serve turkey and vegetable stir-fry over cooked brown rice.

Nutritional Information:
- Calories: 400
- Protein: 30g
- Carbohydrates: 40g
- Fat: 15g

---

4. Lentil and Vegetable Curry

Ingredients:
- 1 cup dried green lentils, rinsed and drained
- 2 cups vegetable broth
- 1 onion, chopped

- 2 cloves garlic, minced
- 1 tbsp curry powder
- 1 tsp ground cumin
- 1 tsp ground turmeric
- 1 can (14 oz) diced tomatoes
- 2 cups mixed vegetables (e.g., bell peppers, zucchini, cauliflower)
- 1 can (14 oz) coconut milk
- Salt and pepper to taste
- Cooked brown rice, for serving

Instructions:
1. In a large pot, combine lentils, vegetable broth, onion, garlic, curry powder, cumin, and turmeric. Bring to a boil, then reduce heat and simmer for 20-25 minutes, or until lentils are tender.
2. Stir in diced tomatoes, mixed vegetables, and coconut milk. Simmer for an additional 10 minutes, or until vegetables are tender.
3. Season with salt and pepper.
4. Serve lentil and vegetable curry over cooked brown rice.

Nutritional Information:
- Calories: 350
- Protein: 15g
- Carbohydrates: 50g
- Fat: 10g

---

5. Turkey and Vegetable Skillet

Ingredients:
- 1 lb ground turkey
- 1 tbsp olive oil
- 1 onion, chopped
- 2 cloves garlic, minced
- 2 cups mixed vegetables (e.g., bell peppers, zucchini, corn)
- 1 can (14 oz) diced tomatoes

- 1 tsp Italian seasoning
- Salt and pepper to taste
- Cooked whole wheat pasta, for serving

Instructions:
1. In a large skillet, heat olive oil over medium heat. Add ground turkey and cook until browned.
2. Add onion and garlic to the skillet. Cook, stirring occasionally, until onion is translucent.
3. Stir in mixed vegetables, diced tomatoes, Italian seasoning, salt, and pepper. Simmer for 10-15 minutes, or until vegetables are tender.
4. Serve turkey and vegetable mixture over cooked whole wheat pasta.

Nutritional Information:
- Calories: 400
- Protein: 30g
- Carbohydrates: 40g
- Fat: 15g

---

6. Veggie-Packed Chili

Ingredients:
- 1 tbsp olive oil
- 1 onion, chopped
- 2 cloves garlic, minced
- 2 bell peppers, diced
- 2 carrots, diced
- 1 zucchini, diced
- 1 can (14 oz) diced tomatoes
- 1 can (14 oz) kidney beans, drained and rinsed
- 1 can (14 oz) black beans, drained and rinsed
- 2 cups vegetable broth
- 2 tbsp chili powder

- 1 tsp cumin
- Salt and pepper to taste

Instructions:
1. In a large pot, heat olive oil over medium heat. Add onion and garlic and cook until softened.
2. Add bell peppers, carrots, and zucchini to the pot. Cook, stirring occasionally, until vegetables are tender.
3. Stir in diced tomatoes, kidney beans, black beans, vegetable broth, chili powder, cumin, salt, and pepper. Bring to a simmer and cook for 20-30 minutes, stirring occasionally.
4. Serve veggie-packed chili hot.

Nutritional Information:
- Calories: 350
- Protein: 15g
- Carbohydrates: 60g
- Fat: 5g

---

7. Lemon Herb Baked Cod

Ingredients:
- 4 cod fillets
- 2 tbsp olive oil
- 1 lemon, juiced and zested
- 2 cloves garlic, minced
- 1 tsp dried thyme
- 1 tsp dried rosemary
- Salt and pepper to taste

Instructions:
1. Preheat oven to 400°F (200°C).
2. Place cod fillets on a baking sheet lined with parchment paper.

3. In a small bowl, combine olive oil, lemon juice, lemon zest, garlic, thyme, rosemary, salt, and pepper.
4. Brush the olive oil mixture over the cod fillets.
5. Bake in the preheated oven for 12-15 minutes, or until the fish is opaque and flakes easily with a fork.
6. Serve lemon herb baked cod hot.

Nutritional Information:
- Calories: 300
- Protein: 30g
- Carbohydrates: 2g
- Fat: 18g

---

8. Vegetarian Stuffed Bell Peppers

Ingredients:
- 4 bell peppers, halved and seeded
- 1 cup cooked quinoa
- 1 can (14 oz) black beans, drained and rinsed
- 1 can (14 oz) diced tomatoes
- 1 cup corn kernels
- 1 tsp cumin
- 1 tsp chili powder
- Salt and pepper to taste
- 1/2 cup shredded cheddar cheese (optional)

Instructions:
1. Preheat oven to 350°F (175°C).
2. In a large bowl, combine cooked quinoa, black beans, diced tomatoes, corn, cumin, chili powder, salt, and pepper.
3. Fill each bell pepper half with the quinoa mixture. Place stuffed bell peppers in a baking dish.

4. Cover the baking dish with foil and bake in the preheated oven for 25-30 minutes, or until the bell peppers are tender.
5. If desired, sprinkle shredded cheddar cheese over the stuffed bell peppers during the last 5 minutes of baking.
6. Serve vegetarian stuffed bell peppers hot.

Nutritional Information:
- Calories: 350
- Protein: 15g
- Carbohydrates: 60g
- Fat: 5g

---

9. Vegetable and Tofu Stir-Fry

Ingredients:
- 1 tbsp sesame oil
- 1 block (14 oz) firm tofu, drained and cubed
- 2 cups mixed vegetables (e.g., bell peppers, broccoli, snap peas, carrots)
- 2 cloves garlic, minced
- 2 tbsp soy sauce
- 1 tbsp hoisin sauce
- 1 tsp ginger, grated
- Cooked brown rice, for serving

Instructions:
1. Heat sesame oil in a large skillet or wok over medium-high heat.
2. Add cubed tofu and cook until browned on all sides.
3. Add mixed vegetables and garlic to the skillet. Cook, stirring frequently, until vegetables are tender-crisp.
4. In a small bowl, whisk together soy sauce, hoisin sauce, and grated ginger. Pour sauce over tofu and vegetables. Stir to combine.
5. Serve vegetable and tofu stir-fry over cooked brown rice.

Nutritional Information:
- Calories: 400
- Protein: 20g
- Carbohydrates: 45g
- Fat: 15g

---

10. Lentil and Mushroom Shepherd's Pie

Ingredients:
- 1 cup dried green lentils, rinsed and drained
- 2 cups vegetable broth
- 1 onion, chopped
- 2 cloves garlic, minced
- 8 oz mushrooms, chopped
- 1 tsp dried thyme
- 1 tsp dried rosemary
- Salt and pepper to taste
- 4 cups mashed potatoes (prepared)
- 1/4 cup grated Parmesan cheese

Instructions:
1. Preheat oven to 375°F (190°C).
2. In a large pot, combine lentils, vegetable broth, onion, garlic, mushrooms, thyme, rosemary, salt, and pepper. Bring to a boil, then reduce heat and simmer for 20-25 minutes, or until lentils are tender.
3. Transfer lentil mixture to a baking dish. Spread mashed potatoes over the top.
4. Sprinkle grated Parmesan cheese over the mashed potatoes.
5. Bake in the preheated oven for 25-30 minutes, or until the top is golden brown.

Nutritional Information:
- Calories: 350

- Protein: 15g
- Carbohydrates: 50g
- Fat: 10g

---

11. Baked Chicken and Vegetable Casserole

Ingredients:
- 4 boneless, skinless chicken breasts
- 2 cups mixed vegetables (e.g., carrots, peas, corn)
- 1 can (10.5 oz) cream of chicken soup
- 1/2 cup Greek yogurt
- 1/2 cup shredded cheddar cheese
- Salt and pepper to taste
- 1 cup cooked brown rice

Instructions:
1. Preheat oven to 375°F (190°C).
2. Place chicken breasts in a baking dish. Season with salt and pepper.
3. In a bowl, combine mixed vegetables, cream of chicken soup, Greek yogurt, and shredded cheddar cheese. Pour mixture over chicken breasts.
4. Cover baking dish with foil and bake in the preheated oven for 30 minutes.
5. Remove foil and bake for an additional 15 minutes, or until chicken is cooked through and top is bubbly.
6. Serve chicken and vegetable casserole over cooked brown rice.

Nutritional Information:
- Calories: 400
- Protein: 35g
- Carbohydrates: 30g
- Fat: 15g

---

12. Veggie-Packed Spaghetti Squash Boats

Ingredients:
- 1 medium spaghetti squash
- 1 tbsp olive oil
- 1 onion, chopped
- 2 cloves garlic, minced
- 1 bell pepper, chopped
- 1 zucchini, chopped
- 1 cup cherry tomatoes, halved
- 1 can (15 oz) chickpeas, drained and rinsed
- 1 tsp dried oregano
- 1/2 tsp red pepper flakes
- Salt and pepper to taste
- 1/4 cup grated Parmesan cheese

Instructions:
1. Preheat oven to 400°F (200°C).
2. Cut spaghetti squash in half lengthwise and remove seeds. Place squash halves cut side down on a baking sheet. Bake for 30-40 minutes, or until tender.
3. In a large skillet, heat olive oil over medium heat. Add onion and garlic. Cook until softened.
4. Add bell pepper, zucchini, cherry tomatoes, and chickpeas to the skillet. Cook, stirring occasionally, until vegetables are tender.
5. Use a fork to scrape the spaghetti squash into strands. Add squash strands to the skillet. Stir in oregano, red pepper flakes, salt, and pepper.
6. Divide the mixture evenly between the squash halves. Sprinkle with grated Parmesan cheese.
7. Return squash boats to the oven and bake for an additional 10 minutes, or until heated through.

Nutritional Information:
- Calories: 350
- Protein: 12g

- Carbohydrates: 50g
- Fat: 12g

---

13. Mediterranean Chickpea Salad

Ingredients:
- 1 can (15 oz) chickpeas, drained and rinsed
- 1 cucumber, diced
- 1 bell pepper, diced
- 1/2 red onion, thinly sliced
- 1/4 cup chopped fresh parsley
- 1/4 cup chopped fresh mint
- 1/4 cup crumbled feta cheese
- 2 tbsp olive oil
- 2 tbsp lemon juice
- 1 clove garlic, minced
- Salt and pepper to taste

Instructions:
1. In a large bowl, combine chickpeas, cucumber, bell pepper, red onion, parsley, mint, and feta cheese.
2. In a small bowl, whisk together olive oil, lemon juice, garlic, salt, and pepper.
3. Pour dressing over chickpea mixture. Toss to combine.
4. Serve Mediterranean chickpea salad chilled or at room temperature.

Nutritional Information:
- Calories: 350
- Protein: 15g
- Carbohydrates: 45g
- Fat: 15g

---

14. Turkey and Quinoa Stuffed Bell Peppers

Ingredients:
- 4 bell peppers, halved and seeds removed
- 1 cup cooked quinoa
- 1 lb ground turkey
- 1 onion, chopped
- 2 cloves garlic, minced
- 1 can (14 oz) diced tomatoes
- 1 tsp dried oregano
- 1/2 tsp red pepper flakes
- Salt and pepper to taste
- 1/2 cup shredded mozzarella cheese

Instructions:
1. Preheat oven to 375°F (190°C).
2. Place bell pepper halves in a baking dish.
3. In a large skillet, cook ground turkey, onion, and garlic until turkey is browned and cooked through. Drain any excess fat.
4. Stir in cooked quinoa, diced tomatoes, oregano, red pepper flakes, salt, and pepper.
5. Spoon turkey and quinoa mixture into bell pepper halves. Sprinkle with shredded mozzarella cheese.
6. Cover baking dish with foil and bake in the preheated oven for 25-30 minutes, or until peppers are tender.
7. Remove foil and bake for an additional 5 minutes, or until cheese is melted and bubbly.

Nutritional Information:
- Calories: 400
- Protein: 30g
- Carbohydrates: 30g
- Fat: 15g

---

8. Snack Recipes

1. Hummus and Veggie Sticks

Ingredients:
- 1/2 cup hummus
- 1 carrot, cut into sticks
- 1 cucumber, cut into sticks
- 1 bell pepper, cut into strips

Instructions:
1. Serve hummus with carrot sticks, cucumber sticks, and bell pepper strips for dipping.

Nutritional Information:
- Calories: 150
- Protein: 5g
- Carbohydrates: 20g
- Fat: 7g

---

2. Greek Yogurt Parfait

Ingredients:
- 1/2 cup Greek yogurt
- 1/4 cup granola
- 1/4 cup mixed berries (e.g., strawberries, blueberries, raspberries)

Instructions:
1. Layer Greek yogurt, granola, and mixed berries in a glass or bowl.

Nutritional Information:
- Calories: 200
- Protein: 15g

- Carbohydrates: 30g
- Fat: 5g

---

3. Almond Butter and Banana Slices

Ingredients:
- 2 tbsp almond butter
- 1 banana, sliced

Instructions:
1. Spread almond butter on banana slices.

Nutritional Information:
- Calories: 200
- Protein: 5g
- Carbohydrates: 25g
- Fat: 10g

---

4. Rice Cake with Avocado

Ingredients:
- 1 rice cake
- 1/4 avocado, mashed
- Sprinkle of sea salt and black pepper

Instructions:
1. Spread mashed avocado on rice cake. Sprinkle with sea salt and black pepper.

Nutritional Information:
- Calories: 100

- Protein: 2g
- Carbohydrates: 15g
- Fat: 5g

---

5. Trail Mix

Ingredients:
- 1/4 cup almonds
- 1/4 cup cashews
- 1/4 cup dried cranberries
- 1/4 cup dark chocolate chips

Instructions:
1. Mix all ingredients together.

Nutritional Information:
- Calories: 300
- Protein: 7g
- Carbohydrates: 25g
- Fat: 20g

---

6. Apple Slices with Peanut Butter

Ingredients:
- 1 apple, sliced
- 2 tbsp peanut butter

Instructions:
1. Spread peanut butter on apple slices.

Nutritional Information:
- Calories: 200

- Protein: 4g
- Carbohydrates: 25g
- Fat: 10g

---

7. Cottage Cheese with Pineapple

Ingredients:
- 1/2 cup low-fat cottage cheese
- 1/2 cup diced pineapple

Instructions:
1. Serve cottage cheese topped with diced pineapple.

Nutritional Information:
- Calories: 150
- Protein: 15g
- Carbohydrates: 20g
- Fat: 2g

---

8. Whole Grain Crackers with Cheese

Ingredients:
- 6 whole grain crackers
- 1 oz cheddar cheese, sliced

Instructions:
1. Serve whole grain crackers with cheddar cheese slices.

Nutritional Information:
- Calories: 200
- Protein: 8g

- Carbohydrates: 20g
- Fat: 10g

---

9. Roasted Chickpeas

Ingredients:
- 1 can (15 oz) chickpeas, drained and rinsed
- 1 tbsp olive oil
- 1 tsp smoked paprika
- 1/2 tsp garlic powder
- 1/2 tsp cumin
- Salt to taste

Instructions:
1. Preheat oven to 400°F (200°C).
2. Pat chickpeas dry with a paper towel and place on a baking sheet.
3. Drizzle with olive oil and sprinkle with smoked paprika, garlic powder, cumin, and salt. Toss to coat.
4. Roast in the preheated oven for 20-25 minutes, or until crispy.

Nutritional Information:
- Calories: 200
- Protein: 8g
- Carbohydrates: 30g
- Fat: 5g

---

10. Kale Chips

Ingredients:
- 1 bunch kale, stems removed and leaves torn into bite-sized pieces
- 1 tbsp olive oil

- 1/2 tsp sea salt

Instructions:
1. Preheat oven to 300°F (150°C).
2. In a large bowl, toss kale leaves with olive oil and sea salt.
3. Spread kale leaves in a single layer on a baking sheet.
4. Bake in the preheated oven for 20-25 minutes, or until crispy.

Nutritional Information:
- Calories: 150
- Protein: 5g
- Carbohydrates: 15g
- Fat: 8g

---

9. Dessert Recipes

-1. Banana Oat Cookies

Ingredients:
- 2 ripe bananas, mashed
- 1 cup rolled oats
- 1/4 cup chopped nuts (e.g., walnuts, almonds)
- 1/4 cup chocolate chips
- 1/2 tsp cinnamon
- 1/2 tsp vanilla extract

Instructions:
1. Preheat oven to 350°F (175°C).
2. In a bowl, combine mashed bananas, oats, chopped nuts, chocolate chips, cinnamon, and vanilla extract.
3. Drop spoonfuls of the mixture onto a baking sheet lined with parchment paper.
4. Bake for 15-20 minutes, or until cookies are golden brown.

Nutritional Information:
- Calories: 100
- Protein: 2g
- Carbohydrates: 15g
- Fat: 4g

---

2. Baked Apples

Ingredients:
- 2 apples, cored
- 2 tbsp chopped nuts (e.g., pecans, almonds)
- 1 tbsp honey
- 1/2 tsp cinnamon

- 1/4 cup water

Instructions:
1. Preheat oven to 375°F (190°C).
2. In a bowl, mix chopped nuts, honey, and cinnamon.
3. Stuff each apple with the nut mixture.
4. Place stuffed apples in a baking dish and pour water into the dish.
5. Bake for 30-40 minutes, or until apples are tender.

Nutritional Information:
- Calories: 200
- Protein: 2g
- Carbohydrates: 30g
- Fat: 10g

---

3. Chocolate Avocado Pudding

Ingredients:
- 2 ripe avocados, peeled and pitted
- 1/4 cup cocoa powder
- 1/4 cup honey or maple syrup
- 1/2 tsp vanilla extract
- Pinch of salt
- Optional toppings: berries, shredded coconut, chopped nuts

Instructions:
1. In a food processor, blend avocados, cocoa powder, honey or maple syrup, vanilla extract, and salt until smooth.
2. Refrigerate for at least 30 minutes before serving.
3. Serve topped with berries, shredded coconut, or chopped nuts if desired.

Nutritional Information:
- Calories: 200

- Protein: 3g
- Carbohydrates: 25g
- Fat: 12g

---

4. Greek Yogurt with Honey and Almonds

Ingredients:
- 1 cup Greek yogurt
- 2 tbsp honey
- 2 tbsp sliced almonds

Instructions:
1. Divide Greek yogurt into serving bowls.
2. Drizzle honey over the yogurt.
3. Sprinkle sliced almonds on top.

Nutritional Information:
- Calories: 200
- Protein: 15g
- Carbohydrates: 20g
- Fat: 8g

---

5. Fruit Salad

Ingredients:
- 1 cup mixed berries (e.g., strawberries, blueberries, raspberries)
- 1 orange, peeled and segmented
- 1 banana, sliced
- 1/2 cup grapes, halved

Instructions:
1. Combine all fruits in a bowl.
2. Serve as is or with a dollop of Greek yogurt on top.

Nutritional Information:
- Calories: 150
- Protein: 2g
- Carbohydrates: 35g
- Fat: 1g

---

6. Chia Seed Pudding

Ingredients:
- 1/4 cup chia seeds
- 1 cup almond milk
- 1 tbsp honey or maple syrup
- 1/2 tsp vanilla extract
- Fresh berries for topping

Instructions:
1. In a bowl, mix chia seeds, almond milk, honey or maple syrup, and vanilla extract.
2. Refrigerate for at least 2 hours, or overnight, until thickened.
3. Serve topped with fresh berries.

Nutritional Information:
- Calories: 200
- Protein: 5g
- Carbohydrates: 25g
- Fat: 10g

---

7. Frozen Banana Bites

Ingredients:
- 2 ripe bananas, peeled and cut into slices
- 1/4 cup peanut butter
- 1/4 cup dark chocolate chips

Instructions:
1. Spread peanut butter on banana slices and sandwich them together to form bites.
2. Place banana bites on a baking sheet lined with parchment paper.
3. Melt dark chocolate chips in the microwave or over a double boiler.
4. Drizzle melted chocolate over banana bites.
5. Freeze for at least 1 hour before serving.

Nutritional Information:
- Calories: 150
- Protein: 3g
- Carbohydrates: 20g
- Fat: 8g

---

8. Coconut Macaroons

Ingredients:
- 2 cups shredded coconut
- 1/2 cup almond flour
- 1/4 cup honey or maple syrup
- 1/4 cup coconut oil, melted
- 1 tsp vanilla extract
- Pinch of salt
- Optional: dark chocolate for dipping

Instructions:
1. Preheat oven to 350°F (175°C) and line a baking sheet with parchment paper.
2. In a bowl, mix shredded coconut, almond flour, honey or maple syrup, melted coconut oil, vanilla extract, and salt until well combined.
3. Scoop mixture into small mounds on the baking sheet.
4. Bake for 10-12 minutes, or until golden brown.
5. Let cool completely. Optional: dip cooled macaroons in melted dark chocolate.

Nutritional Information:
- Calories: 150
- Protein: 2g
- Carbohydrates: 10g
- Fat: 12g

---

9. Baked Cinnamon Apples

Ingredients:
- 2 apples, cored and sliced
- 1 tbsp honey or maple syrup
- 1/2 tsp cinnamon
- 1/4 cup chopped nuts (e.g., pecans, walnuts)

Instructions:
1. Preheat oven to 350°F (175°C).
2. Place apple slices in a baking dish.
3. Drizzle honey or maple syrup over apple slices and sprinkle with cinnamon.
4. Bake for 20-25 minutes, or until the apples are tender.
5. Serve topped with chopped nuts.

Nutritional Information:
- Calories: 150
- Protein: 2g
- Carbohydrates: 25g
- Fat: 6g

---

10. Frozen Yogurt Bark

Ingredients:
- 2 cups Greek yogurt
- 2 tbsp honey or maple syrup
- 1/2 cup mixed berries (e.g., strawberries, blueberries, raspberries)
- 1/4 cup granola

Instructions:
1. Line a baking sheet with parchment paper.
2. In a bowl, mix Greek yogurt and honey or maple syrup.
3. Spread yogurt mixture evenly onto the prepared baking sheet.
4. Sprinkle mixed berries and granola over the yogurt.
5. Freeze for at least 2 hours, or until firm.
6. Break into pieces before serving.

Nutritional Information:
- Calories: 200
- Protein: 10g
- Carbohydrates: 30g
- Fat: 5g

---

10. Smoothie and Juice Recipes

1. Berry Blast Smoothie

Ingredients:
- 1/2 cup mixed berries (e.g., strawberries, blueberries, raspberries)
- 1/2 banana
- 1/2 cup spinach
- 1/2 cup almond milk
- 1 tbsp chia seeds
- 1/2 tsp honey or maple syrup (optional)

Instructions:
1. Combine all ingredients in a blender.
2. Blend until smooth.
3. Pour into a glass and enjoy!

Nutritional Information:
- Calories: 150
- Protein: 5g
- Carbohydrates: 25g
- Fat: 5g

---

2. Green Goodness Juice

Ingredients:
- 1 cucumber
- 2 celery stalks
- 1 green apple
- 1/2 lemon, peeled
- 1 inch piece of ginger

Instructions:
1. Wash all produce.
2. Juice all ingredients in a juicer.
3. Stir well and serve over ice.

Nutritional Information:
- Calories: 100
- Protein: 2g
- Carbohydrates: 25g
- Fat: 1g

---

3. Tropical Paradise Smoothie

Ingredients:
- 1/2 cup pineapple chunks
- 1/2 banana
- 1/2 cup mango chunks
- 1/2 cup coconut milk
- 1/2 cup orange juice
- 1 tbsp shredded coconut

Instructions:
1. Combine all ingredients in a blender.
2. Blend until smooth.
3. Pour into a glass and enjoy!

Nutritional Information:
- Calories: 200
- Protein: 2g
- Carbohydrates: 40g
- Fat: 5g

---

4. Carrot-Orange Juice

Ingredients:
- 4 carrots
- 2 oranges, peeled
- 1 inch piece of ginger

Instructions:
1. Wash all produce.
2. Juice all ingredients in a juicer.
3. Stir well and serve over ice.

Nutritional Information:
- Calories: 150
- Protein: 3g
- Carbohydrates: 35g
- Fat: 1g

---

5. Creamy Berry Smoothie

Ingredients:
- 1/2 cup mixed berries (e.g., strawberries, blueberries, raspberries)
- 1/2 banana
- 1/2 cup Greek yogurt
- 1/2 cup almond milk
- 1 tbsp honey or maple syrup (optional)

Instructions:
1. Combine all ingredients in a blender.
2. Blend until smooth.
3. Pour into a glass and enjoy!

Nutritional Information:
- Calories: 200
- Protein: 10g
- Carbohydrates: 35g
- Fat: 5g

---

6. Blueberry Banana Smoothie

Ingredients:
- 1/2 cup blueberries
- 1/2 banana
- 1/2 cup spinach
- 1/2 cup almond milk
- 1 tbsp almond butter
- 1/2 tsp honey or maple syrup (optional)

Instructions:
1. Combine all ingredients in a blender.
2. Blend until smooth.
3. Pour into a glass and enjoy!

Nutritional Information:
- Calories: 200
- Protein: 5g
- Carbohydrates: 30g
- Fat: 8g

---

7. Citrus Sunshine Juice

Ingredients:
- 2 oranges, peeled

- 1 grapefruit, peeled
- 1 lemon, peeled
- 1 inch piece of turmeric
- 1 inch piece of ginger

Instructions:
1. Wash all produce.
2. Juice all ingredients in a juicer.
3. Stir well and serve over ice.

Nutritional Information:
- Calories: 150
- Protein: 3g
- Carbohydrates: 35g
- Fat: 1g

---

8. Peanut Butter Banana Smoothie

Ingredients:
- 1/2 banana
- 1 tbsp peanut butter
- 1/2 cup Greek yogurt
- 1/2 cup almond milk
- 1 tbsp honey or maple syrup (optional)

Instructions:
1. Combine all ingredients in a blender.
2. Blend until smooth.
3. Pour into a glass and enjoy!

Nutritional Information:
- Calories: 250
- Protein: 15g

- Carbohydrates: 30g
- Fat: 10g

---

9. Green Detox Juice

Ingredients:
- 1 cucumber
- 2 celery stalks
- 1 green apple
- 1/2 lemon, peeled
- 1 handful of kale

Instructions:
1. Wash all produce.
2. Juice all ingredients in a juicer.
3. Stir well and serve over ice.

Nutritional Information:
- Calories: 100
- Protein: 3g
- Carbohydrates: 25g
- Fat: 1g

---

10. Chocolate Banana Protein Smoothie

Ingredients:
- 1/2 banana
- 1 tbsp cocoa powder
- 1/2 cup Greek yogurt
- 1/2 cup almond milk
- 1 scoop chocolate protein powder

Instructions:
1. Combine all ingredients in a blender.
2. Blend until smooth.
3. Pour into a glass and enjoy!

Nutritional Information:
- Calories: 300
- Protein: 30g
- Carbohydrates: 35g
- Fat: 5g

---

11. Supplements and Prostate Health

Supplements can play a role in supporting prostate health, especially when combined with a balanced diet and healthy lifestyle. While it's important to consult with a healthcare provider before starting any new supplement regimen, here are some supplements that are commonly used to support prostate health:

1. Saw Palmetto: Saw palmetto is a popular herbal supplement used to support prostate health. It may help reduce symptoms of an enlarged prostate, such as frequent urination and nighttime urination.

2. Beta-Sitosterol: Beta-sitosterol is a plant sterol that may help improve urinary symptoms associated with benign prostatic hyperplasia (BPH), a non-cancerous enlargement of the prostate gland.

3. Pygeum: Pygeum is an herbal supplement derived from the bark of the African plum tree. It has been used traditionally to support prostate health and may help reduce urinary symptoms associated with BPH.

4. Zinc: Zinc is an essential mineral that plays a role in prostate function and health. Some studies suggest that zinc supplementation may help reduce the risk of developing prostate cancer.

5. Vitamin D: Vitamin D deficiency has been linked to an increased risk of prostate cancer. Taking a vitamin D supplement may help support prostate health, especially in individuals with low vitamin D levels.

6. Fish Oil: Fish oil supplements, which are rich in omega-3 fatty acids, may help reduce inflammation and support overall prostate health.

7. Selenium: Selenium is a trace mineral that plays a role in antioxidant defense. Some studies suggest that selenium supplementation may help reduce the risk of prostate cancer, especially in men with low selenium levels.

8. Lycopene: Lycopene is a powerful antioxidant found in tomatoes and other red fruits and vegetables. Some studies suggest that lycopene supplementation may help reduce the risk of prostate cancer.

It's important to note that while supplements can be beneficial, they should not be used as a substitute for a healthy diet and lifestyle. It's always best to consult with a healthcare provider before starting any new supplement regimen, especially if you have underlying health conditions or are taking medications.

- Recommended Dosages and Considerations

When taking supplements for prostate health, it's important to follow recommended dosages and consider individual health factors. Here are some general guidelines:

1. Saw Palmetto: Typical dosages range from 320 mg to 640 mg daily, standardized to contain 85-95% fatty acids and sterols. It's best to take saw palmetto with food to enhance absorption.

2. Beta-Sitosterol: Dosages vary, but a common recommendation is 60-130 mg per day, taken with meals.

3. Pygeum: Typical dosages range from 50 mg to 200 mg per day, standardized to contain 13% total sterols. Pygeum is often taken in divided doses with food.

4. Zinc: The recommended daily intake of zinc for adult men is 11 mg. Excessive zinc intake can interfere with copper absorption, so it's important not to exceed the recommended dosage.

5. Vitamin D: The recommended daily intake of vitamin D varies based on age and other factors. For adults, the recommended dietary allowance (RDA) is 600-800 IU per day.

6. Fish Oil: Dosages vary depending on the concentration of omega-3 fatty acids in the supplement. A common recommendation is 1-2 grams of combined EPA and DHA per day.

7. Selenium: The recommended daily intake of selenium for adults is 55 mcg. It's important not to exceed the tolerable upper intake level of 400 mcg per day, as high doses can be toxic.

8. Lycopene: Dosages vary, but a common recommendation is 10-30 mg per day. Lycopene supplements are often taken with meals to enhance absorption.

When taking supplements, it's important to consider potential interactions with medications and other supplements. Always consult with a healthcare provider before starting any new supplement regimen, especially if you have underlying health conditions or are taking medications.

12. Lifestyle Tips for Prostate Health

- Exercise and Physical Activity Recommendations

Regular physical activity is beneficial for prostate health. Here are some exercises and activities that can help support prostate health:

1. Aerobic Exercise: Engage in moderate-intensity aerobic exercise for at least 150 minutes per week, or vigorous-intensity aerobic exercise for 75 minutes per week. Aerobic activities such as walking, jogging, cycling, swimming, or dancing can help improve cardiovascular health and overall well-being.

2. Strength Training: Incorporate strength training exercises into your routine at least two days per week. Focus on exercises that target major muscle groups, such as squats, lunges, push-ups, and weightlifting. Strength training can help improve muscle strength, bone density, and metabolism.

3. Pelvic Floor Exercises (Kegels): Pelvic floor exercises, also known as Kegels, can help strengthen the muscles that support the bladder, bowel, and prostate. To do Kegels, tighten the muscles used to stop the flow of urine, hold for a few seconds, and then relax. Repeat this exercise several times throughout the day.

4. Yoga or Pilates: Consider practicing yoga or Pilates, which can help improve flexibility, balance, and core strength. These forms of exercise can also help reduce stress and promote relaxation, which is beneficial for overall health.

5. Tai Chi: Tai Chi is a gentle form of martial arts that combines slow, flowing movements with deep breathing and meditation. Tai Chi can help improve balance, flexibility, and mental well-being.

6. Sports and Recreational Activities: Engage in sports or recreational activities that you enjoy, such as tennis, golf, swimming, or hiking. These activities can help you stay active and fit while having fun.

7. Walking: Walking is a simple and effective form of exercise that can be easily incorporated into your daily routine. Aim to walk briskly for at least 30 minutes a day to help improve cardiovascular health and maintain a healthy weight.

8. Cycling: Cycling is another low-impact exercise that can be beneficial for prostate health. Whether you prefer riding outdoors or using a stationary bike indoors, cycling can help improve cardiovascular fitness and leg strength.

It's important to consult with a healthcare provider before starting any new exercise regimen, especially if you have underlying health conditions or concerns. Listen to your body and choose activities that are enjoyable and sustainable for you. By staying active and incorporating regular physical activity into your routine, you can help support prostate health and overall well-being.

- Stress Management and Sleep Hygiene

Stress management and good sleep hygiene are important components of maintaining overall health, including prostate health. Here are some tips for managing stress and improving sleep quality:

Stress Management:
1. Mindfulness Meditation: Practice mindfulness meditation to help reduce stress and promote relaxation. Focus on the present moment and let go of worries about the past or future.
2. Deep Breathing Exercises: Practice deep breathing exercises to help calm the mind and body. Inhale deeply through your nose, hold for a few seconds, and exhale slowly through your mouth.
3. Yoga or Tai Chi: Engage in yoga or Tai Chi, which can help reduce stress and improve flexibility and balance.

4. Regular Exercise: Stay physically active, as exercise can help reduce stress and improve mood. Aim for at least 150 minutes of moderate-intensity aerobic exercise per week.
5. Healthy Lifestyle Choices: Maintain a healthy lifestyle by eating a balanced diet, staying hydrated, limiting alcohol and caffeine intake, and avoiding tobacco use.

Sleep Hygiene:
1. Consistent Sleep Schedule: Go to bed and wake up at the same time every day, even on weekends, to regulate your body's internal clock.
2. Comfortable Sleep Environment: Create a comfortable sleep environment that is cool, dark, and quiet. Use earplugs or a white noise machine if needed.
3. Limit Screen Time: Avoid screens (e.g., smartphones, tablets, computers) at least an hour before bed, as the blue light can interfere with your body's natural sleep-wake cycle.
4. Relaxation Techniques: Practice relaxation techniques such as progressive muscle relaxation or guided imagery before bed to help calm your mind and prepare for sleep.
5. Limit Stimulants: Avoid stimulants such as caffeine and nicotine close to bedtime, as they can interfere with your ability to fall asleep.
6. Regular Exercise: Regular physical activity can help improve sleep quality. However, avoid vigorous exercise close to bedtime, as it may interfere with your ability to fall asleep.

By incorporating these stress management techniques and sleep hygiene practices into your daily routine, you can help reduce stress, improve sleep quality, and support overall prostate health. If you continue to experience significant stress or sleep disturbances, consider speaking with a healthcare provider for further guidance and support.

13. Resources and Support for Prostate Cancer Patients

- Organizations and Websites for Further Information

1. Prostate Cancer Foundation (PCF) - The PCF is a leading organization dedicated to funding research into the prevention, diagnosis, and treatment of prostate cancer. Their website provides information on prostate cancer, treatment options, and support resources. (https://www.pcf.org/)

2. American Cancer Society (ACS) - The ACS is a nationwide organization dedicated to eliminating cancer as a major health problem. Their website offers information on prostate cancer, including prevention, early detection, treatment, and support services. (https://www.cancer.org/)

3. Us TOO International Prostate Cancer Education and Support Network - Us TOO is a nonprofit organization that provides support, education, and advocacy for men with prostate cancer and their families. Their website offers resources, support group information, and educational materials. (https://www.ustoo.org/)

4. Prostate Cancer UK - Prostate Cancer UK is a charity that provides information, support, and research funding for prostate cancer. Their website offers resources for patients, families, and healthcare professionals. (https://prostatecanceruk.org/)

5. National Cancer Institute (NCI) - The NCI is part of the National Institutes of Health (NIH) and is the U.S. government's principal agency for cancer research. Their website provides information on prostate cancer, treatment options, clinical trials, and support services. (https://www.cancer.gov/)

6. Movember Foundation - The Movember Foundation is a global charity that raises awareness and funds for men's health issues, including prostate

cancer. Their website offers resources and information on prostate cancer prevention, early detection, and treatment. (https://us.movember.com/)

Support Groups for Prostate Cancer Patients and Families

1. Us TOO International Prostate Cancer Support Groups - Us TOO offers support groups for men with prostate cancer and their families. Their support groups provide a safe and confidential environment to share experiences and receive emotional support. (https://www.ustoo.org/Find-a-Support-Group)

2. Cancer Support Community - The Cancer Support Community offers support groups for cancer patients and their families, including those affected by prostate cancer. Their support groups are facilitated by licensed professionals and provide emotional support and coping strategies. (https://www.cancersupportcommunity.org/)

3. American Cancer Society (ACS) Support Groups - The ACS offers online and in-person support groups for cancer patients and their families, including those affected by prostate cancer. Their support groups provide a forum to share experiences, ask questions, and receive support. (https://www.cancer.org/treatment/support-programs-and-services.html)

4. Local Hospitals and Cancer Centers - Many hospitals and cancer centers offer support groups for prostate cancer patients and their families. These support groups may be facilitated by healthcare professionals and provide a supportive environment to discuss concerns and receive information. Contact your local hospital or cancer center for more information.

These organizations and support groups can provide valuable information, resources, and emotional support for prostate cancer patients and their families.

14. Conclusion

Encouragement for Making Positive Dietary Changes

Embarking on a journey to improve your diet and nutrition can be challenging, but it is also incredibly rewarding. Every step you take towards making positive dietary changes is a step towards better health and well-being. Here are some words of encouragement to support you along the way:

1. Believe in Yourself: Believe that you have the strength and determination to make positive changes in your diet and nutrition. You have the power to take control of your health and make choices that will benefit you in the long run.

2. Take it One Step at a Time: Making dietary changes can feel overwhelming, but remember that progress is made one step at a time. Start by making small, achievable changes and gradually build on them over time.

3. Celebrate Your Successes: Celebrate your successes, no matter how small. Whether it's choosing a healthy snack over a sugary treat or adding more vegetables to your meals, every positive choice you make is a step in the right direction.

4. Focus on the Benefits: Keep your focus on the benefits of making dietary changes, such as improved energy levels, better mood, and reduced risk of chronic diseases. Visualize the positive impact these changes will have on your health and well-being.

5. Seek Support: Don't be afraid to seek support from friends, family, or healthcare professionals. Having a support system can make it easier to stay motivated and accountable.

6. Be Kind to Yourself: Remember that change takes time, and it's okay to have setbacks along the way. Be kind to yourself and treat yourself with compassion as you work towards your goals.

7. Stay Positive: Stay positive and optimistic about your ability to make lasting changes. You have the power to create a healthier future for yourself, and every positive choice you make is a step in the right direction.

Remember, making positive dietary changes is an investment in your health and well-being. Stay committed, stay focused, and believe in yourself. You have the strength and determination to create a healthier, happier you.

In conclusion, "The Prostate Cancer Diet and Nutrition Handbook for Men Over 50" aims to empower and educate readers on the vital role that diet and nutrition play in managing prostate health. From understanding the importance of key nutrients to implementing lifestyle changes that promote overall well-being, this book serves as a comprehensive guide for navigating the complexities of prostate cancer.

By incorporating the principles outlined in this book into your daily life, you can take proactive steps towards improving your prostate health and overall quality of life. Remember, small changes can lead to significant results, and by prioritizing your health and well-being, you are taking a proactive approach to managing prostate cancer.

We hope that this book has provided you with valuable insights, practical tips, and a sense of empowerment as you embark on your journey towards better prostate health. Together, we can work towards a future where prostate cancer is no longer a threat, and all men can enjoy optimal health and vitality.

Thank you for allowing us to be a part of your journey towards prostate health. Wishing you health, happiness, and a fulfilling life ahead.